Introducing the First Book in the

Clover Series of Tender Teaching™

In the story, Clover is afraid of what her friends might do or say when she gets head lice.

I believe that learning more about head lice will make it less scary.

Clover's entertaining story will help you and those you know learn about head lice in a fun way!

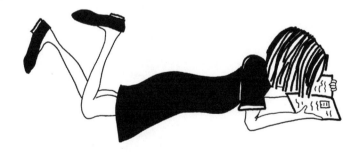

Thank you to my family for your honesty and humor.

"The only one who didn't get lice was the dog. Why? Because we don't have a dog!" - Comedian

Clover Series of Tender Teaching: Book #1

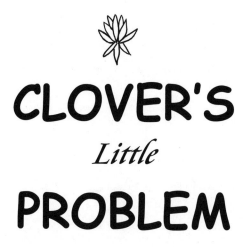

CLOVER'S
Little
PROBLEM

Written and Illustrated by

B. L. Dawson

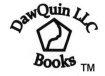

Contact the author/publisher at info@dawquin.com or
DawQuin LLC, P.O. Box 1800, Troy, MI 48099

Dawson, B. L. (Barbara L.)

Clover's little problem / written and illustrated by B.L. Dawson.

  p. : ill. ; cm. -- (Clover series of tender teaching ; bk. #1)

Includes bibliographical references.
  Summary: This is the story of Clover, a third grade girl who gets head lice, her treatment at home, reactions from friends, and dealing with the school bully, all from her perspective. The reader is educated about head lice, its causes, symptoms, diagnosis and treatment. Included are detailed appendices and a list of resources.
  Interest age level: 008-012.

  ISBN: 978-0-9842787-0-1 (hardcover)
  ISBN: 978-0-9842787-1-8 (pbk.)

1. Pediculosis--Juvenile fiction.   2. Lice--Juvenile fiction.   3. Pediculosis--Fiction.   4. Lice--Fiction. I. Title.

PZ7.D39 Cl 2010
[Fic]   2010920367

Manufactured by Thomson-Shore, Dexter, MI (USA); RMA566TB027, March, 2010

CONTENTS

The Story

Appendices

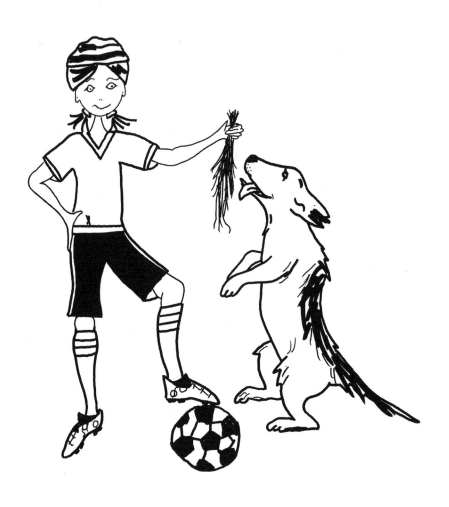

Chapter 1

The Haircut

One of the most difficult things I ever did turned out to be one of the best things ever. I did it last year. I cut my hair! You're thinking, "So big deal." Well, for me it was. I had the longest and most beautiful hair in the whole wide world. I know this because everybody was always telling me, "Clover, you have beautiful hair."

So why did I cut it? The answer is wigs. Yes, wigs. I cut it to help other kids who have lost their hair because of some sickness. I went from being scared of cutting my hair to being so, so happy.

My brand new haircut looked great. My hair isn't short, but it isn't long anymore either. It is sort of medium. The haircut lady styled it so I look like a famous movie star. Everybody loved it, and some of my friends even went out and did the same thing.

The hair that was cut off mine will make a beautiful wig for a sick kid. I hope they make a girl wig out of it. I'd hate to see them waste it for a boy, but I guess boys are allowed to have nice hair too.

Rob in my class has nice hair. I would never tell him that because he thinks he is the greatest at everything. He would just think that his hair is better than mine, and it is not.

Now that I have this problem he will probably be teasing me when I go back to school tomorrow. I can hear him now. "Clover, you should have cut all your hair off last year!"

He will probably be playing soccer at recess. He is good at soccer. I have to admit that even though I do not think he has the greatest hair.

I will stay off the soccer field so Rob will not make fun of me. Teams play every recess, and we keep score for the month. We called our team the Bears. Rob's team was the Rhinos. My team lost to Rob's team two times. We lost because I gave some other kids a try at goalkeeper. Last month we won with me back in goal. The Bears need another win this month to tie the series.

I like to play goalkeeper. It is my favorite position. Most kids are afraid of the ball. Not me.

Rob can kick really hard but last recess I blocked him six times. That is even more reason to stay away, because he will be out to get me back for blocking him. If he can't beat me, he may tease me in front of everybody.

My team probably won't want me around them anyway. Who wants to play with a kid that has head lice?

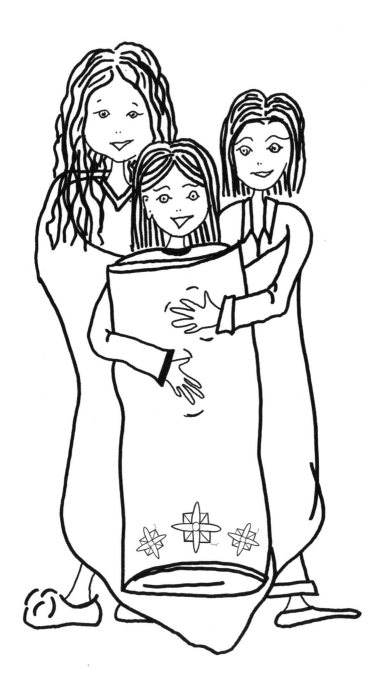

Chapter 2

All in the Family

We all got head lice: me and both my sisters. Daisy is the oldest and she still has long, beautiful hair. We couldn't talk her into cutting it for the sick kids or even after the lice came to our house.

My other older sister is Violet. She cut her hair when I did. It looked good but not as good as mine.

My mom named us all after flowers. She even named the dog after a part of a flower, Petal. She loves her flower garden. She calls it "her" garden even though Dad does most of the work in it.

I think Dad doesn't have enough hair to get lice. His hair is so thin that it is almost not hair at all but mostly baldness. Mom says that doesn't matter and that everyone gets checked every day.

They found lice on Violet then called me down to the school office. There was one tiny little egg on my hair and so I got sent home with Violet. How can one tiny egg cause such big problems?

Ms. Sandra, the office lady, says that you usually don't see the actual lice because they are fast and hide from the light. That is why they check for nits.

The head lice eggs are called "nits." Violet's hair had a lot of nits.

Me and my sisters like to cuddle together on a super huge pillow under a blanket and watch TV. The lice or louse probably ran from Violet's head to mine when we were touching heads.

If it is just one, you call it a louse. Like mouse is one and mice are more than one. Just change the "M" to "L" and you have lice or louse. Both a louse and a mouse can be a pain if you get them in your house.

Even without TV time it would have been easy to share lice with my sisters because we share everything, including a room, clothes, coats, hats, brushes, and hair bands. We are close like that.

My sister Daisy who was in the older school got lice too. Mom picked her up after getting us so that Daisy wouldn't "share it with her friends."

Daisy's face turned white as a ghost when she saw us. She must have thought something really bad had happened. It sort of did.

Mom explained to her about the lice right in front of the office staff. Daisy looked like she wanted to crawl into a hole. She had to be worried her friends would find out. Most likely she was more concerned about what this meant for her beautiful hair.

Now that all of us were going home, Mom had more help for the hardest parts.

 Good to Know!

It is not always necessary to miss school. You may discover head lice and treat it without ever missing school.

Lice and nits are usually found in dark warm places on our heads, like the crown area, behind our ears, and near the neck.

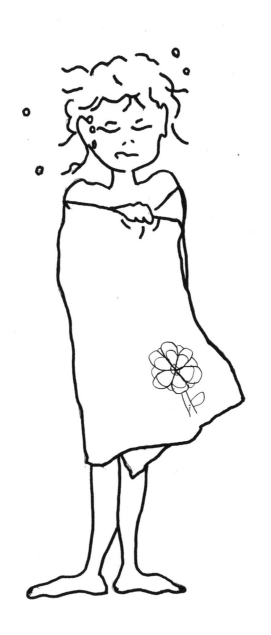

Chapter 3

The Shampoo

We all had our hair washed with special shampoo, especially Violet.

I had to because of the one nit Ms. Sandra found on me. That probably meant that there was or had been a female louse in my hair.

Females are girls. Males are boys. A female louse can lay *at least* 3 nits a day for 30 days. I'm good at math. That means more than 90 eggs in a month or a lot of itching. I can see how this lice thing could get out of control very fast. Fortunately, not all of the eggs will hatch into babies.

Mom had checked Daisy's hair immediately when we got home from school and found three nits. Because Mom had fallen asleep with Daisy the night before, she assumed she had lice too.

Mom likes to cuddle and talk with us in our beds. We really enjoy talking at night for some reason. I always end up telling her stuff about me or my friends. Lots of times she falls asleep in my bed too.

Sometimes I crawl in with her. Dad will carry me back to my own room. He doesn't even try to carry Mom back to her room. Just once I would like to see him try. It would be good to see for a laugh or two.

Our family also talks at dinner. We go around the table and tell about our day. You better think about something to say. If you don't then Mom will come back to you until she gets some piece of information out of you.

And don't just say anything because Dad follows it with one hundred questions so you better know how to answer them. I actually enjoy our dinners together.

I did not enjoy the hair washing. In fact, it was horrible. I normally like a good shampoo. It feels good to rub my head. This time we had to sit with the medicated soap on our heads for a long time. Dad called it "pesticides," which are chemicals to kill bugs, but the bottle said "shampoo."

Sometimes adults forget kids can read. My Mom still spells words around my birthday time, thinking she is keeping my gift a surprise. Whether she says it or spells it, I can figure it out. Just like I can figure out not to use this special shampoo without a parent.

"Never use this stuff without your mother or me. It is not a normal shampoo. It can hurt you if used wrong!" Dad was very serious. Mom put the little bit we didn't use in the top of the cabinet where we cannot reach.

We actually saw dead lice when we rinsed off Violet's head. Violet thought it was neat. She likes bugs and science and stuff. I do too, but not as much as Violet.

The dead lice were small, about the size of a rice grain, and black or brown. Mom says they can be light gray to dark tan or black. It is hard to tell black or brown on something that small. Dad even has trouble with socks. Sometimes he wears one black with one brown sock. He doesn't notice until he is at work under the bright lights. I don't think it bothers him much.

The stuff they put on my head bothered me. I hoped it wasn't destroying my beautiful hair. It was going to be hard enough to go back and face my friends at school. It would be even worse with bad hair!

As it turned out my hair smelled a little different but didn't look unusual. The shampoo was only part of it. There was more that had to be done before going back to school.

 Good to Know!

Itching is not always a sign of head lice. Some people are allergic to the saliva from the mouth of the lice and this makes them itch. Others never itch.

Just because your head itches does not mean you have head lice. There are many other reasons for an itchy head.

Head lice and body lice are different. Body lice are associated with unclean people. However, head lice can affect clean and dirty persons.

Chapter 4

Nit Picking

When I was young, tangles would get bad in my hair. It would take my mom a long time to get all the tangles out. I complained the entire time.

Right after the lice shampoo, Mom combed every strand of hair on my head. It reminded me of when I had tangles in my hair. It didn't hurt but it took long, and I complained the entire time.

The special lice comb caught nits that the shampoo missed. Mom would take a small bit of hair and comb through it making sure she started close to our scalp and she pulled all the way down until the end of our hair.

After each pull she wiped any lice eggs off and threw them in a plastic bag. When all done, she sealed the bag and put it in the garbage.

It took a long time to comb my hair and even more time for Daisy. I bet she wished she had donated some of her hair to those sick kids.

Dad's hair went the fastest and then he combed Mom's hair. One time, we all helped check Mom's hair. I have to admit it was fun telling her to "sit still" like she always says to us.

Apparently, the nits are attached to the hair with really strong "glue." This is good and bad.

The good part is it helps to tell if you have lice or normal stuff. Normal hair stuff is leftover shampoo or conditioner, dirt, oil, and dandruff.

Dandruff is the white flaky stuff in our hair. They can look almost the same but the dandruff will move easy, whereas the nits stick to the hair.

Sometimes there are hair shafts that can be mistaken for nits. I think hair shafts are just buildup of that normal stuff in our hair. They wrap all around the hair strand.

Lucy in my class always seems to have stuff that is not normal in her hair. Lucy likes art. Almost every day she brings in something she made for our teacher.

She never plays soccer at recess. She likes to make sculptures in the sand box. In winter, she will use the snow. She is really good at art but not so good at clean up.

I sit next to her at school and can always see paint, sparkles, or glitter in her hair. I wonder what her pillow looks like at home. I also wonder what Ms. Sandra would say looking in Lucy's hair.

Ms. Sandra uses a flashlight and magnifying glass to check for nits. She says it is easier to see the different shapes.

Nits are shaped like a tear or water drop. They appear yellow, white, grayish, or brown color. They can be the size of a pinhead- that's small. Mother lice stick them very close to our head on a strand of hair. The heat from our head helps keep their babies warm. The nits stay stuck to the piece of hair as our hair grows. The nits are stuck very tight on the hair and this is the bad part. They are hard to get off.

We got to watch TV while Mom examined our hair for nits. Normally we are not allowed to watch TV on school nights. Dad says we should be focused on practicing piano and doing homework, not on TV.

We do get to watch it on weekends. However, I usually miss when I have soccer games. I like

Saturday morning cartoons, but no more watching on our super huge pillow. We had to bag that during the clean-up.

Good to Know!

Nit or lice combs have very narrow spaces between the teeth to catch the tiny lice eggs. Normal combs will not work.

Nits found close to our heads are probably alive. Nits found over ½ inch away are probably dead or hatched.

It is <u>very</u> important to check and comb for 21 days. Medicated shampoos will NOT kill all the nits and lice.

Chapter 5

Home

Mom should not sing. Or dance. Or do anything musical for that matter. In fact, we told her so. However, in the privacy of our own home we give her a little creative space. In other words, we let her sing and dance all she wants provided none of our friends are visiting. She really loves to "rock the house" while cleaning.

Cleaning. Only this time Mom really meant it. Usually I can pick-up a few dirty clothes and shove the rest under my made-up bed. Not this time. Mom bent down to check under our beds with her big butt swaying to the music that was blaring throughout the house.

We all joined in, singing and twirling, while we put everything dirty into bags, including the mattress covers. Mom decided to "get it over with" and go to the Laundromat. We could have washed it all at

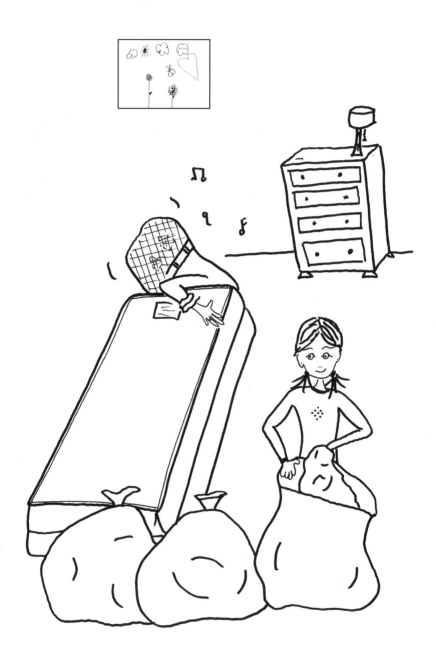

home but Mom said since she had so many helpers we could each take a machine at the mat.

All of our pillows, sheets, blankets, coats, and hats went into the laundry bags. The clean clothes stayed in our drawers.

Our stuffed animals or plush toys went into a different bag. It was a black plastic bag. Mom tied it tight so nothing could get in or out and put it out of the way.

Our super huge TV pillow was too big for a washing machine or dryer so Daisy and Violet sealed it in a bag, too.

We cannot open them for three whole weeks and by that time any lice will be dead. I hope Dad doesn't take them out with the garbage by mistake. I made a big sign so he wouldn't: **"NOT GARBAGE- VALUABLE ANIMALS INSIDE!"**

If the weather had been colder we could have put the bags outside to freeze overnight. Lice do not like it real cold or real hot. Apparently, the best temperature for lice is on top of my head.

Mom vacuumed the house. She vacuumed the rug in front of the TV, all the couches, and even all the bed mattresses. She sang the entire time – loudly!

She said that she was very happy we are all so close but it would have been easier if only Violet had lice. Then only Violet's area would need cleaning. But since we all got lice everything had to be cleaned.

Well, almost everything. We didn't have to clean our hard toys or books or papers. And we didn't have to clean our desks or tables. We didn't have to clean the garage or kitchen, at least not for the lice. I'm sure Mom or Dad will have us clean those areas later.

Cleaning at home was fun with the music and dancing. It went fast with all of us helping. Everything got shoved in the van, including us. Off we went to the Laundromat with more music playing. No matter how loud it plays Mom always seems to be able to sing louder than the radio.

I didn't want to go. What if my friends saw me? Would they ask why I was not in school? What would I say? Then I realized that all of my friends were probably still at school. If someone was at the

Laundromat, then they wouldn't want me asking any more than I wanted them asking. We could just ignore each other.

More important was what to say when I went back to school. I was also worried about what Mom would say, but she hadn't used the word "Lice" once since entering the Laundromat. Even better, she wasn't singing or dancing either. Maybe she wouldn't gossip with the other parents or teachers about head lice.

It would have been easy to skip the washer and just let the dryer heat work on the lice, but Mom said everything needed a good wash anyway, especially our coats.

Mine was really dirty from playing soccer every recess. The goalkeeper has to dive for the ball a lot.

Daisy's coat was really clean. She takes hours to get ready for school. I think she spends more time doing her hair and trying on outfits than she actually spends at school.

She doesn't play soccer. Her sport is tennis. I think she plays tennis because of the cute outfits.

She has more cute tennis skirts than there are days of the week.

She is actually a good tennis player. She almost always makes it to the finals. A lot of people watch the finals so I guess she does have to look good. I think she likes to win so she can get her picture taken in those cute outfits.

We washed those cute outfits. All day we washed and dried. Mom said we couldn't skip the dryer part because the heat was needed to kill the lice. It was a good idea going to the Laundromat. It would have taken a long time at home with just one machine.

The drive home was quiet. We were all too tired to sing. The radio was off and we drove home in silence.

I thought the Laundromat wasn't so bad after all. We got to eat "junk food" for lunch. Doing laundry had been much better than the hair washing. I didn't want to be at school anyway. In fact, I was more concerned about going back to school than about the silly bugs in my hair.

Good to Know!

Ways to kill lice and nits:
1. *Heat above 130°F for 30 minutes*
2. *Below freezing (32°F) for 24 hours*
3. *Seal in a plastic bag for 21 days*
4. *Soak in isopropyl alcohol or medicated shampoo for one hour.*

*Do **NOT** use these methods on people.*
Use them for such items as clothes, blankets, stuffed animals, and combs.

Remember to get any lice or nits off your everyday combs, brushes, barrettes or hair bands by using one of the ways to kill lice and nits.

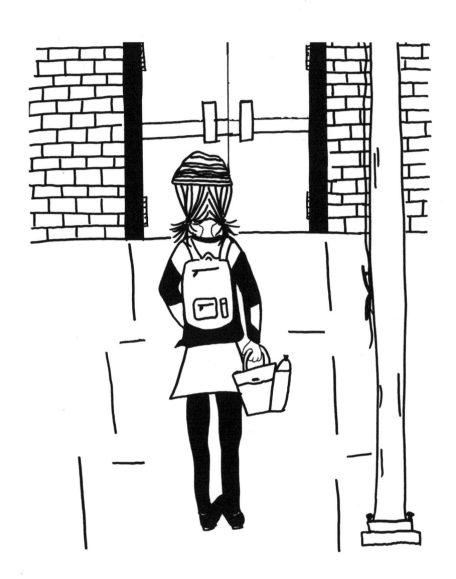

Chapter 6

Going to School

I normally like school. It is fun being with my friends and learning stuff, but now everyone will know about my lice for two reasons.

First, the school knows about our lice. Our class had to put all their coats and stuff in individual plastic bags until the lice are all gone.

So, if you're in a class and suddenly have to put your coat in a plastic bag, you immediately look to see who is not in class that day and that person probably has lice. That person was me.

Daisy's school has lockers but our school just has hooks on the wall so our coats hang touching. I guess the lice can crawl from coat to coat because they are touching but it is not likely that they will crawl through a locker.

The second reason that everybody knew was because Mom called my best friend's parents. We had just come back from a school vacation so I hadn't seen anyone except my two best friends: Dori and Maddy.

They had come over to play on Saturday. It was raining so we stayed inside. We played computer games, a board game, and made chocolate chip cookies.

Mom insisted on calling their parents to give them the "heads up" about my lice. Therefore, everyone would know for sure that I had lice.

I normally sat with Dori on the bus. I was afraid she wouldn't want to sit with me. Why take the chance of getting lice?

Mom says head lice don't jump, hop, or fly. They crawl really well in hair but not as good in other places. If Dori and I are just sitting next to each other without touching, the lice probably won't crawl really fast from me to her. I didn't know if Dori knew that.

Anyway, that day Mom drove me and Violet to school. Usually I like when Mom drives us because we don't have to get ready as early for the bus. Not this time. Mom took us straight to the office so Ms. Sandra could check our hair before class.

I wouldn't like Ms. Sandra's job. All the sick kids go to her and she calls their parents to come get them. She isn't even a nurse or doctor and she has to deal with sick kids all day.

In one way having lice is not as bad as being sick. My throat and belly don't hurt, no boogers or coughing, and no fever. Lice do not make you sick.

However, if I had been sick, I wouldn't be worried about Maddy and Dori ignoring me or Rob poking fun at me.

My hair checked out good. Ms. Sandra found one nit on Violet that Mom had missed.

I felt like crying even though it was on Violet and not me. What if we had to go home and clean, shampoo, and comb again? What if a classmate saw me go into the office and then go home again? They would know for sure we had really bad lice.

Ms. Sandra let Violet go to school anyway because Mom said that Violet was treated just yesterday. Apparently, it is not good for us to repeat the special shampoos too often.

Ms. Sandra cut the nit out of Violet's hair and sealed it between two pieces of tape before tossing it in the garbage. Just then the principal came into the room. She asked Ms. Sandra if everything looked good.

I was scared. Why? Well, not because Mrs. Rockwood is mean or anything, but she is the principal and the principal is responsible for the entire school. I was afraid she would be mad at us for bringing lice into *her* school.

I was just thinking of how I was going to put the blame on Violet (because we think she got it first) when I realized Mrs. Rockwood was not mad. She even put her hand on our shoulders real assuring and told us to go to class so we would not be late. Mom was still talking to her as Violet and I headed to class.

As we were walking, I looked at Violet and she did not seem worried at all. Violet is in fifth grade and I am in third grade. The classes are separated by the fourth grade rooms, so just before we separated I whispered to her, "Aren't you scared?"

"No, not at all. I've been in this school longer than you and seen a lot of kids that had head lice. Remember last year my best friend Selena had it?"

Violet was very calm and not even whispering. I had forgotten that Selena had it last year. Her hair is very curly. That must have been a major pain to comb.

"Did kids make fun of her?" I asked.

"Maybe, but I didn't. We couldn't hug or read with our heads together so that I wouldn't catch it. We did come up with a super cool handshake instead. Clover, if anyone picks on you, just tell Mrs. Rockwood or your teacher. They know how to handle this stuff."

Then Violet gave me a big hug, my only hug for the rest of the school day. I guess she wasn't scared of getting lice because she already had it. But I think she would have given me a hug anyway because she is that kind of sister.

I watched her trot happily off to class. Now I had to face Rob, Maddy, Dori, and the rest of my class alone.

Good to Know!

Most staff at school cannot diagnose head lice. That means they can 'think' they found head lice but cannot say for sure. Check with a doctor or health care professional to confirm you have lice.

Not all principals, secretaries, or teachers act like the ones in our story. Some may not understand and may act mean or grouchy. It is not your fault. Perhaps they should read this book.

Your parents should tell the school office if you get lice. The school cannot tell anyone that you have lice, but can ask parents to check their children at home. This will help keep lice from spreading back and forth.

It is a good idea to keep long hair pulled back in a pony tail or braids during a head lice outbreak at school.

Chapter 7

Sitting in Front

I walked in just as the bell was ringing. Mr. Boarder was handing out the big plastic bags to all the kids. As soon as he saw me he said, "Clover! Welcome back. Here, take this bag and put your coat and stuff in it. Put your backpack in there too after you take out your lunch, water bottle, and homework. You did do your homework?"

Oh, no! I forgot my homework. With all the cleaning, washing, and combing it completely skipped my mind.

"Mr. Boarder, I forgot to do my homework," I answered in a real quiet voice while looking at my feet.

I could feel the whole class staring at me. They were looking at lice girl who did not do her homework.

Mr. Boarder is a fairly cool teacher. The kids who were never in his class make fun of his name and call him "Boring Boarder," but his class is actually a lot of fun. Unfortunately for me, he is very strict about homework. He does not like it to be messy, wrinkled, or late, for any reason, so I was preparing for the worst.

The worst never came. He just told me, "Clover, please hand it in tomorrow, first thing." That took a load off my mind. I was worried about the late homework and almost forgot about the lice. Now that the homework was not a major issue, lice came back full force to the top of my mind.

I got my stuff out from my backpack and put the rest into the plastic bag. We had to write our names on tape for the bag. I sat down at my desk and arranged things: paper, pencils, and books. Everything was just as I had left them, but I rearranged things anyway because I needed someplace to look with my eyes.

The entire time I had been in class I avoided looking at anyone. I didn't look at Mr. Boarder or any kids, not even Dori. Mr. Boarder called the class to attention. He immediately started talking about math story problems that had multiplication answers.

Everyone was paying attention so I decided to glance over toward where Dori sat. I tried not to move my head too much so nobody would notice me.

She wasn't in her seat! We started out in the back of the room together until we got in trouble for talking too much. Then Mr. Boarder sat us right up in the front row but not next to each other.

Lucy, the artist girl, sat next to me. I had looked right past her to check for Dori but now that Dori wasn't there, Lucy caught my eye. She smiled nicely at me. I smiled back as best I could since I did not feel like smiling, and then took a quick glance at her hair. I could still see sparkles and other art supplies on her head so figured she didn't have lice. If she did have lice, all that stuff would have come out in the shampoo and combing, but it was still there.

Where was Dori? Sick? Maybe she had a dentist appointment today. She is late a lot because she goes to the dentist to get her braces adjusted. Oh no! Maybe she has head lice!

She will be so mad at me. She will think I gave her lice even though it was probably Violet. Violet was playing with me, Dori, and Maddy on Saturday. Maddy! I wonder if she is in class. She has a different teacher. I looked out into the hall. Sometimes I can see them coming and going to gym, music, or library. Nobody was in the hall now.

I would have to wait until recess. The entire third grade takes recess at the same time. Recess! I thought of Rob and soccer. He sits behind me. I didn't want to risk a glance backwards so I just pretended to pay attention to Mr. Boarder, but really I was thinking about recess. Was Rob in class today? How bad would he pick on me? Would my team even want me to play goalkeeper anymore? Would I see Maddy on the playground?

 Good to Know!

It is normal to worry about what our friends think. Sometimes even our best friends say or do something that upsets us.

Lice can be difficult on a friendship. You may be ignored, teased, and play dates may even be cancelled. Your friends may not know that they hurt your feelings. Tell them. They may not know how to react. Teach them about head lice.

Your true friends will still be there for you!

Chapter 8

Facing Recess

"Class, get your coats out of your bags for recess." Mr. Boarder was giving out instructions. I stood up and turned around. There he was, Rob. He was pushing another boy who was pushing back while trying to beat each other to their bags.

Normally, I am in a big hurry to go outside and play. Not today. I walked slowly and looked down at my feet so that nobody would notice me, because I just didn't want to be teased about having lice. I figured I would go slowly, the soccer game would start without me, and then I would find Maddy.

Maddy doesn't play soccer. She doesn't like any sports. Actually, I think she does but maybe is afraid of not being good. She watches me and Dori play sports a lot.

My plan was working except for one thing. Maddy was watching soccer today. In order to talk with her, I'd have to go by the soccer field. I took a deep breath and got up my nerve to go over to her.

As soon as she saw me this sad look fell on her face. I thought something was wrong with her then realized the sad look was for me. I just wanted to be treated normal and not draw attention. Her sad look of pity didn't help.

We each said "Hey," then she went on to ask me, "Are you OK?"

Like I had some complicated surgery or someone died. I guess I shouldn't be mad at her. She was just trying to be my friend. Friends are supposed to care about each other. But when I said, "Fine," I blurted it out a little rude. I immediately apologized and told her I was just tired and wished this had never happened. She seemed fine with that.

Just then Rob came over. He immediately began. "So do you or Dori have bugs in your head? Or is it both of you? I didn't think there was anything in your head that even a bug would want."

It hurt even though I had expected it from him. I couldn't think of a comeback when Maddy spoke up.

"That head of hers must have something in it since she is good enough to block you," she exclaimed.

That's when my team came over and asked- no,

begged- me to play goalkeeper. It sure was nice to be wanted: bugs and all.

First, I thanked Maddy and made sure she was fine with me leaving her to go play. She said to get in goal because yesterday was a bad soccer day and our team was down by two points. Of course, she wants our team to win because we are best of friends.

I blocked all of Rob's shots that day, so he was mad at me. He stopped teasing me about lice, though.

Stella, a player on my team, tried to give me a hug after I blocked a really hard shot, but I remembered the lice and instead stuck my hand up to give her a high five. Stella is always hugging. I'm glad she is not in Mr. Boarder's class.

 Good to Know!

It seems like everyone knows a bully. Something like head lice can bring out the worst in them. Talk with your parents, teacher, or another adult about ideas for dealing with bullies.

Remember to hold your head high and walk with confidence. There is nothing wrong with you!

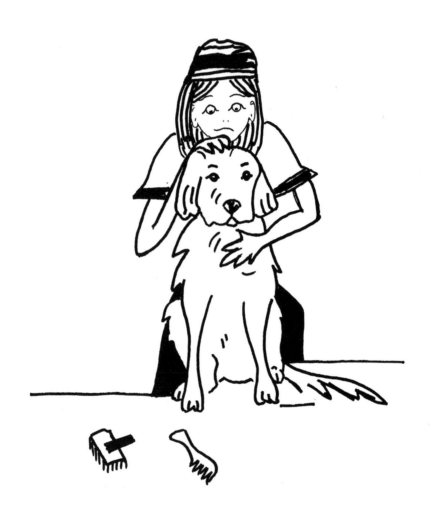

Chapter 9

Across the School

I was glad Maddy was still my friend. She didn't seem to care about head lice.

I rode the bus home sitting next to Violet. I would have sat with Maddy, but she rides a different bus. When I got home, Mom took our coats and hats to be washed- AGAIN! "Just in case." We snacked on a handful of blueberries and a cheese stick. Then Mom checked our hair for nits- AGAIN! When it wasn't our turn, we did homework in our rooms. By the time we finished Dad was home and we ate dinner.

Mom asked, as usual: "How was everyone's day?"

Violet spoke up. "Six kids in my class got lice: Sunita, Sophia, Emily, Hamm, Bruce, and me."

That was four girls and two boys. They all have different hair. Sunita has very long, thick black hair. I think her parents are from India.

Sophia has short black hair. I've heard her and Selena talk in Spanish on the bus. I bet they do great in Spanish class.

Emily has completely different hair from all the rest of the kids. It is red and curly.

Hamm is new to our school. His English is not good. He just came from Korea. He has thick black hair.

The other boy, Bruce, has short, light brown hair. His sister in first grade has very blond hair and also got the lice. I had to laugh. Bruce is Rob's brother. What if Rob got lice from his brother or sister?

Mom explained, "When you girls went to class, Mrs. Rockwood told me that 15 kids were out of school because of lice. She couldn't tell me who, but said at least one kid in every grade. She sent home a note in your backpacks warning parents that lice were found at school. The note went out to the entire school, instead of just the infected classes. Because so many kids have head lice, Mrs. Rockwood felt everyone should be aware. She recommends all parents check their kids every night at home."

"Did she say who got it first?" I asked.

"No, Clover. Mrs. Rockwood can't talk about specific cases. Everyone has a right to privacy. Besides, we may never know who got it first. You and Violet may have got it at school or someplace else. It could have come from a public place, trying on clothes at the store, from a relative or friend's house. Lice have been around for as long as we know and are good at survival and finding warm heads."

Just then it hit me. "Mom! We didn't shampoo and comb Petal!"

Petal is a mutt dog and has a blend of different colors in her thick fur. Petal was definitely in the same places as us. She even likes to lie with us on the floor. I think that is why we always watch TV from the floor. Mom doesn't allow any dog on the furniture or even in the bedrooms. Petal is a great dog. She sleeps in a dog bed just outside our bedroom doors.

Mom said, "We don't have to worry about Petal. Pets don't get our head lice. Anyway, Petal had a bath today because she came in as muddy as your jacket after playing soccer at recess."

Daisy asked, "So why did we have to clean her dog bed at the laundry mat?"

Mom replied, "Because it needed it."

Violet asked, "What do dogs have that we don't to keep lice away?" Dad smiled at that very good question, but nobody knew the answer.

I had to ask. "Mom, did I give lice to Dori?"

"We do not know, Clover. Maybe. Her Mom called and Dori definitely has it. Her Mom treated her with olive oil instead of the special shampoo we used. Apparently, Dori has very sensitive skin and her mother was afraid the lice shampoo would give her chemical burns."

Daisy was laughing. "Olive oil. Did they fry it with garlic first like we do for pasta sauce? I bet her hair is very shiny now. It is probably as shiny as a plastic doll."

Mom gave her the look which means "be nice". Then Dad spoke up. "When I was a kid we would shave our heads when we got lice."

Daisy was appalled. Her smile turned to a frown and she asked, "Even the girls?"

"No, but the girls usually got a very short haircut. And mayonnaise."

This was typical Dad. He usually asked a hundred questions at dinner, especially if we gave short answers. Now we had to ask a hundred questions to get answers from him. He says it is good to ask questions. It shows that you're thinking. So we all asked at the same time, "Mayonnaise?"

"Yes, some people think that the mayonnaise suffocates the lice. When I was a kid, our doctor recommended it. That's what he used."

Daisy commented, "Lice were around even way back then!"

Dad just kept talking. "Mayonnaise, like olive oil, helps to make the hair slick so the lice comb goes through easily. It is difficult to wash out the oil. Mayonnaise has a lot of oil in it."

Mom broke in because she was still thinking about Daisy's comments. "You know, Daisy. Shampoo takes the oil out of our hair. Not only the dirty oil, but our hair's *natural* oil too. Conditioner is an attempt to put that oil back. I bet Dori's hair is very soft and healthy looking now."

That did it. Daisy was now requesting our next treatment be with olive oil. We have to treat our hair again. That way we will get any lice that just hatched from a nit we may have missed. I would like to put a little garlic in Daisy's olive oil to see what that does to her hair.

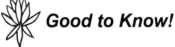 **Good to Know!**

Yes, it is true many people use olive oil for lice. There are many treatments like this. They are called alternative treatments because not a lot of scientific research has been done. However, they may still work.

Lice have been around as long as people remember. They are good at adapting, which is why getting rid of them is difficult.

The nits will hatch 7 to 11 days after being laid. That is why a second hair treatment is always a necessary precaution.

Any person can get head lice, but not our pets.

Your parents or your friends' parents may get grouchy when head lice come home. Remember they may just be tired from the cleaning and such. Try helping. It may make it easier on them.

Chapter 10

Real Friendship

I was afraid that Dori was mad at me. She probably knew I gave her the lice. We needed to talk. I decided to call her after dinner. Her mom, Mrs. Hancock, answered the telephone and started asking how we were all doing and how school went and a hundred other questions. Parents are always fishing for information even if it is not their own kid. Mom says it's her job. Mrs. Hancock finally put Dori on the phone.

"Hello."

"Hey Dori, how are you doing?"

"OK." She sounded sad. Maybe she didn't want to talk to me. I wasn't going to stop so easy, though.

"We missed you at school today. We are down by two points." Dori played on my team at recess.

"Was Rob there?" I guess she dreaded seeing him just as much as I had.

"Yes, he was there. He made fun of us catching lice but Maddy shut him up for us. Maddy doesn't have lice but Rob's brother and sister do. Wouldn't it be funny if Rob got it too?"

Dori laughed at that thought. I supposed this was a good time to say sorry for giving her lice. When I said "sorry," she said "sorry "at the same time.

"Why are you saying 'Sorry'?" I asked.

"Because I probably gave your family lice. My cousin has it, and I was at her house before I went to your house." She sounded like she didn't want to give that piece of information out. I realized she was just as scared as me. Afraid of being the one to give her friends lice. Afraid of being teased, especially by Rob.

"I thought we gave it to you. Mom says it is hard to tell who got it first." I told her how nobody in our family was mad at her, or anybody else for that matter. That seemed to make Dori feel better.

I asked her to sit with me on the bus the next day. She said her mom was driving her because she wanted to be there when Ms. Sandra re-checked her hair. Mrs. Hancock was currently in the car putting sheets over the seats.

My mom had put sheets on the couches and big chairs. She said it was easier to throw a sheet in the wash than the whole couch. We hadn't thought about the car seats.

Dori said we could ride home together on the bus. I told her to think of a special handshake to use instead of hugging. Dori likes to hug as much as Stella on our team. We both felt much better after talking. I was glad I called her.

Just over a week later Mom treated our hair with olive oil. Daisy acted like it was some movie star glamour hair treatment. We had to leave the olive oil in a lot longer than the medicated shampoo. We put shower caps and sweat bands on our heads to keep the oil from making a mess.

Actually, I didn't see any big difference. It was still a pain to sit and have my hair combed. The thrill of TV on a weeknight was wearing off. Even though Mom hadn't found a louse or nit all week, she still needed to comb again and then continue checking for the whole three weeks. She didn't want to "go through this again."

47

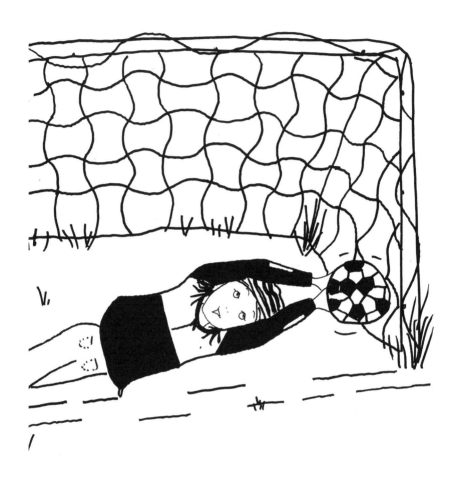

Chapter 11

The Game

I had more important things on my mind than lice. There was only one day left in the month. The score was tied. If a team was ahead after the morning recess then the game was over. But if it was still a tie then the afternoon recess would be a shootout.

That morning was very cold. I kept jumping up and down to stay warm in the goal. We did not let them score at morning recess. Unfortunately, they kept us from scoring also. So there was going to be a shootout that afternoon.

At lunch everyone was talking about it. Everyone but Rob. It was strange. He was usually loud. I expected him to be exchanging comments, back and forth, about who is the better team, but he was just sitting quietly a little off to himself. Come to think about it, he had been quiet all day. The lunch bell rang.

We had art class before the final recess. Our art teacher was absent. The sub gave us fat markers and big sheets of paper. We could draw anything we wanted. Most kids made posters for our soccer shootout.

Lucy, who never paid any attention to soccer, made an excellent poster for the Bears. It said, "Go Bears Go!" and she drew a bear kicking a soccer ball past a rhino. The bear was a girl and the rhino was a boy. The actual goalkeeper for the Rhino's was Samantha, a girl. I hope she didn't see Lucy's poster. She does have short hair like a boy but she definitely looks like a girl. Regardless, Lucy really is a good artist. I hoped her poster would come true and the Bears would win.

All of third grade rushed out to recess. This is normal. However, this time everyone went to the soccer field, even Lucy.

It was exciting. Maddy started a cheer for the Bears and Sara started one for the Rhinos. Everyone had brought their posters from art class. Mr. Boarder and the other third grade teachers were even watching.

It was a little warmer than in the morning, but still cool. Everyone was wearing warm coats and bouncing a little while rubbing hands together to keep warm.

Both teams lined up at midfield. Three at a time would come up to take turns trying to score. Then the goalkeepers would switch and three players from the other team would try scoring. This would continue until all the players had tried to score. The team with the most points would win. This put a lot of pressure on the goalkeeper. I actually like it. I play better under pressure.

Samantha and I shook hands and wished each other good luck. She went into goal first. Dean, Dori, and James kicked from our team. Dean and Dori scored! Bears winning 2-0. My turn. Faith, Noel, and Jerry kicked at me. Nobody scored.

We kept switching in goal. Samantha didn't let anyone else score. Our team was done kicking. We had 2 points. I had also let in 2 points so the score was 2-2, a tie. Three people were left for the Rhinos: Shelby, Xavier, and Rob.

I was nervous. All I had to do was block three shots and it would be a tie. We hadn't talked about what to do if the shootout was a tie. It had never happened before. In fact, this was the first time we ever needed a shootout. Even though I had no idea what would happen if the Bears and Rhinos tied, I still didn't want to lose. I just had to block the last three kicks.

First, Shelby lined up about eight steps behind the ball. She is left footed, which is a little more difficult for the goalkeeper. I watched her eyes for a clue as to where she would kick. Her eyes told me nothing.

I got down in my ready position: hands out, legs spread, and knees bent- ready to leap like a cat. Shelby ran up. At the last minute she looked up and I saw her eye look toward one corner of my goal. I leaped that way as she kicked the ball. I put my arms out over my head as far as they would stretch, then let myself fall toward the ground at the corner. The ball hit my fingers. I held them as straight as I could and the ball bounced out back toward the field. Save!

The crowd went crazy. There was cheering and waving of the posters. I immediately began to prepare for the next kicker, Xavier. I brushed the dirt off me and got into the ready position in the center of the goal. I was somewhat relieved it was Xavier's turn to kick. He usually kicks directly at the center of the goal, which is exactly where I was standing. The only bad thing is that he kicks hard and in the air, so if I miss it with my hands then the ball thumps me in the belly.

I had on my heavier jacket because today was chilly, so that would help cushion the blow. I decided not to take any chances just in case he did not hit directly in the center. This was too important to our team. I paid real close attention to him as he ran up to the soccer ball and kicked.

He did exactly as I thought and I caught it with just a little smack to my belly. Again the crowd went crazy!

Last kicker, Rob. He is the best soccer player in our grade and maybe even the best in the school. I have blocked him a lot, but he has also scored a lot.

Every month he scores almost all the points for the Rhinos team.

I had to concentrate. I blocked out the crowd so it was just Rob and the soccer ball and me and my goal. I was ready.

Rob ran up to the ball. I saw him look at the corner of the goal toward my right. I leaped that way with my arms out. Wait! He kicked toward the other corner. I tried to stop and go the other way but just ended up falling as the ball went into the empty space at the other end of the goal. Rob had tricked me and won the game for the Rhinos.

He stood there with his arms straight over his head in a show of victory. The crowd ran out to him, patted his back, cheered, and hugged each other. Then we all lined up to shake hands and say "good game" to each other.

Maddy and Dori tried to comfort me. I was surprised that I was not too upset. I guess because I tried my hardest and got beat by a very good soccer player. The next time I may just as well block him. The only thing I dreaded was the teasing I was expecting from Rob.

Chapter 12

Again?

The next day was snowy. A heavy snow as high as my boot. I was surprised we had school but Dad said most of the snow fell early last night so the trucks had time to clear the roads before morning. None of the kids could wait until recess. We were all fidgeting in our chairs so finally Mr. Boarder announced, "First big snow, we should be outside!"

We all ran to our bags and pulled out coats, hats, scarves, and gloves. Most of the kids started playing with the snow when we got outside. Nobody went to the soccer field, not even Rob. I expected him to be playing in the snow. Actually, throwing snowballs, but all kids know not to throw snowballs at school. It is an automatic visit to Mrs. Rockwood's office.

Rob was sitting alone, looking real sad, on a bench where the teachers usually sat. I didn't want to be teased about losing the shootout but went over to him anyway.

I stood there and said, "Hey, nice score yesterday."

"Thanks." He looked up trying to smile but actually looked even more sad.

"What's wrong?" I asked.

"Nothing. Why?" said Rob.

"Because you won for the Rhinos and you're not even happy about it."

"That was easy." I saw the old Rob's mischievous smile as he looked up, but just for a second, then he got sad again.

"Easy? If that was so easy then what is so difficult that makes you so unhappy?"

"Nothing." He was quiet and didn't look up so I decided he wanted to be alone. I had just turned to walk away when he said, "Promise you won't tell anyone?"

I turned back and sat beside him on the bench. He was looking at me. "Promise," I said.

He looked into his lap quiet again. I said, "What is it?"

"Never mind." He didn't look up.

I wasn't going to beg for information. This was Rob, the guy that always teased me. It wasn't like he was my close friend. We just happened to both like soccer and got stuck in the same class together. Dori, Maddy, and I always listen to each other's problems. That's what friends do. Where were Rob's friends?

I started getting up to go play, and Rob blurted out, "I have lice!" Then he looked around as if to see if anyone heard and looked at me. I thought he was going to cry. I remembered that this guy was always teasing people. This was my chance to tease him back. Only I didn't feel like it. I had lice only a short time ago. The feelings were still fresh in my mind. I remember being scared of Rob's teasing that first day back. Then it hit me. Rob was scared of being teased. Maybe he knew other kids wanted to pay him back.

I eased back onto the bench and asked, "Since when?"

"The day before our shootout. My dad found it after school. He checks our heads every day because Bruce had it. He found some new ones on me. I shampooed that night and never missed school. That is why we are still bagging our coats."

I hadn't thought about that. I assumed we were still bagging because of Dori and me but our lice had passed. We were bagging because of Rob's lice.

"So you washed with special shampoo, combed your hair, and did laundry?" His coat did look clean.

"Yep," said Rob.

"So what's the problem?" I asked this like it was no big deal, but I remembered lice had been a big deal to me too.

"All those kids were patting my back and hugging me yesterday. I probably gave the whole third grade lice."

"I don't think so, but maybe." Now I was wondering.

"I wanted to stay home but my dad wouldn't let me. I thought of telling everyone but didn't. Then I was going to let you block me so nobody would touch me." He said this like it was his choice whether to score or not and it had nothing to do with my goalkeeping.

Joking a little, I replied, "So it wasn't a good thing for me to let you score the winning point?"

This made him smile. A real smile, not the fake one like earlier. I continued, "You probably gave everyone the flu if you had the sniffles, but I doubt lice. Yesterday was cold and lice do not like cold or light. They were probably hiding close to your head keeping warm. They don't like to run up and down chairs to get from one person to another in class so I don't think they were out watching soccer yesterday. Besides, you just had a hair treatment and they are probably all gone except maybe a nit or two."

"So how do you know so much about lice?" asked Rob.

"Anyone who gets it learns. My mom and the other parents are always talking about how to get rid of lice. Apparently, there are many opinions on the subject."

Rob thought about that for a moment and then challenged, "I bet I can build a bigger snowman."

I was glad he felt better. "You mean 'Lice-man'?"

Rob laughed and said, "Let's build one together."

"OK."

As we got up to build a snowman, Rob said, "Hey Clover, thanks."

"For what?" I asked.

"Not teasing me," said Rob.

"You're welcome," I said. "Bet I can build a bigger snowball."

Rob and I made a huge snowman we didn't finish until second recess. We joked about not putting our hats on the snowman so he wouldn't get lice.

I guess some good things came out of all this lice business. I still kept my true friends, Dori and Maddy, and even made a new one, Rob. All said and done, I think I'd rather have lice than the flu because I didn't miss much school and was still basically healthy. I don't think everyone would agree with me on that, but that is all right.

 Good to Know!

Head lice can return. It may be from the first time or from a completely different source. It is not your fault. Stick to what you just learned and eventually you will be head lice free!

ABOUT HEAD LICE

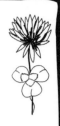

- Head lice are insects.
- Adults are typically 1mm~5mm long.
- A louse may be light gray to dark tan or black.
- Lice do not jump, hop, or fly. They crawl.
- They feed on blood by biting the scalp (like mosquitoes).
- Itching may occur, but not always.
- Head lice are not known to spread any illness or disease (lice will not make you sick).
- A louse is one and lice are more than one.
- A louse lives about 30 days.
- Pediculosis is an infestation of head lice.
- Lice are very fast, hide from light, and usually cannot be seen.
- Their claws are perfect for holding on to our hair but not as good at holding on to thicker objects like rope, carpet or clothing.
- Head lice are different than body lice. It is not necessary to treat other parts of your body if you have head lice.
- Because the insect is so fast, we look for their eggs.
- Head lice eggs are called "nits" (this is where the saying "nit picking," meaning to pick at very small things, came from).
- Nits appear white, yellow, gray, tan, or brown.

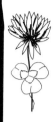

About Head Lice continued...

- *Nits are typically 0.3mm~0.8mm long.*
- *They can be oval or teardrop shaped.*
- *A female louse attaches her nits to individual hairs with strong "glue."*
- *The female may lay 3~6 eggs per day (90~180 eggs per month).*
- *The eggs hatch in 7~11 days.*
- *The eggs need warm temperatures to hatch, like those found on our heads.*
- *Generally speaking, nits found within ¼ inch of the scalp a have a higher probability of being active (alive). If the nit is more than ½ inch away, then it probably already hatched or is not viable (dead).*

HOW TO GET HEAD LICE:

- *Anyone can get it: young, old, poor, rich, clean, dirty.*
- *Head to head contact. (Pets do not get lice.)*
- *Sharing items like combs, brushes, hats, towels, bedding, and hair clips. (Do not share with your BFF.)*
- *Putting your head on infested furniture, rugs, or car seats. (Do not lay your head on the carpet in public places, like the school or library.)*

- *From coats, hats, scarves that had been touching. (Hang your coat separately in public places or keep it next to you.)*

DID YOU KNOW THAT?

- *Under the best of conditions a louse cannot survive more than a few days away from its host (a person's head).*
- *Under normal conditions they probably die within hours off the host.*
- *The egg can survive longer (about a week) away from a host, but when it hatches the louse must eat almost immediately or it will die.*

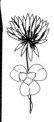

LIFE CYCLE OF A HEAD LOUSE

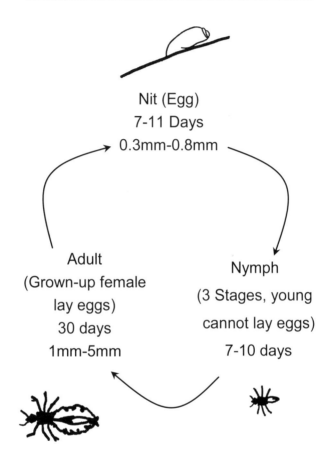

Nit (Egg)
7-11 Days
0.3mm-0.8mm

Adult
(Grown-up female
lay eggs)
30 days
1mm-5mm

Nymph
(3 Stages, young
cannot lay eggs)
7-10 days

(These pictures are a lot bigger than the real thing.)

HOW TO GET RID OF HEAD LICE:

There are many opinions on this subject. Some are based on scientific research, others on personal experience, and still others on what seems like folklore. Review the Resource Section for places to search for information. Following is the author's summary from research and experience. It is not intended to replace the advice or direction offered by your health care provider.

IMPORTANT MESSAGE FOR KIDS !

Always tell your parents if you think you have head lice. Many lice products contain harmful chemicals. The temperatures required to kill lice can burn or cause frost bite.

NEVER TRY TO GET RID OF HEAD LICE YOURSELF.

ALWAYS TELL AN ADULT IF YOU THINK YOU HAVE HEAD LICE.

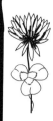

ENVIRONMENT

+ *Lice do not like extremely hot or cold conditions.*

+ *For lice on items like clothes, pillows, or towels (not our heads), wash for at least 10 minutes at 130-140ºF followed by 30 minutes in a dryer at high heat.*

+ *Items that cannot be washed may be sealed in a plastic bag and stored for 21 days or allowed 24 hours in below freezing temperatures.*

+ *It is not necessary to wash all hard surfaces, but do soak (not boil) combs, brushes, and hair accessories in water hotter than 130ºF for 10 minutes or soak them in rubbing alcohol or a medicated shampoo for one hour.*

+ *Vacuum all upholstery, carpets, and bare mattresses.*

+ *It is not necessary to spray or fumigate your house with harmful chemicals.*

+ *Inform others you have been in contact with, i.e. schools, daycare, friends, and family.*

+ *Try not to share items like coats, hats, and brushes and keep your head and hair to yourself.*

HEAD LICE ON OUR HEADS

- *Examine each family member's head daily for three weeks. This is very important or the head lice may and usually do return.*

- *To examine hair, search small sections of hair for nits (eggs). Look close to the scalp for the newer nits. Use a flashlight or magnifying lens to see well. Use a toothpick or finger to try and move the nits. Remember, nits are stuck with strong "glue" and do not move easily. For more details on what to look for see the previous section titled: About Head Lice.*

- *Remove nits (with comb, scissors, or pull out hair strand), seal in a plastic bag, and throw away.*

- *There are many medicated over-the-counter or prescription lice shampoos available. Use these strictly in accordance with label directions. Do not overuse!*

- *There are other treatments marketed that contain "natural" ingredients. Again, use caution and follow directions.*

- *Never use toxic or flammable materials. Never use lindane.*

- *Many of the alternative methods fall under the category of suffocants. Olive oil, mayonnaise, and other oils fall into this group. Suffocants block or obstruct the breathing of lice. Usually multiple*

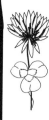

treatments are required. To use: smother your hair and scalp entirely with the chosen product and cover with a shower cap. Some say to leave on overnight while others insist 3-4 hours is enough time. (Use caution if keeping on overnight with children.) Comb with a nit comb, then shampoo, and then comb again! The first combing with the nit comb is to get out the actual lice. The oils usually just slow lice down but do not kill them. The second combing is to get all the nits. Afterward, some parents blow the hair with a heated dryer until completely dry. Little scientific research has been done on these methods. However, the author knows many people who have testified to their effectiveness. That is why Dori was chosen to use the olive oil treatment. It is also the author's opinion that we should always look to minimize our exposure to harmful chemicals.

♦ *With all treatments COMBING IS VERY IMPORTANT. Even the best of chemicals are not 100% effective. Special combs are required that have narrowly spaced teeth. This mechanical pull will help release remaining nits. Remember, their "glue" is very strong. Use the comb, your fingers, or cut* out the individual strand to remove the nits. Otherwise, the lice will come back.

♦ Most products, including combs, are available at your local pharmacy or grocery store.

♦ There are many shampoos that claim to and may actually repel head lice. Many contain herbs or oils that may cause allergic reactions. Use the same precautions as with any product.

♦ Consult your doctor, community health center, or health care provider for the treatment that is right for you and your family.

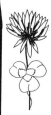

WHAT THE SCHOOL SHOULD DO:

- *Inform the parents that head lice were found in their child's classroom. Request parents to check their children at home.*

- *Respect the privacy of the child and family. Never say who has head lice, only that it was found in a particular classroom or grade.*

- *Separate coats, gloves, scarves, and backpacks that may be touching. Use individual sealed plastic bags for these personal items until the infestation is resolved.*

- *Vacuum carpeted areas daily.*

- *Remove any stuffed animals, pillows, costumes, or plush items from the classroom until the infestation is resolved.*

- *Never make a child feel it is their fault or that they did something wrong by getting head lice.*

- *Teach children not to lie on the carpet, hug, share hats, or touch heads during an infestation.*

- *There is debate about whether the school should administer school-wide head lice checks. Some feel that because it is very common, does not transmit disease, and has probably already spread by the time a case is detected, that the school-wide checks are not necessary. Others feel that by checking after long breaks from school and immediately before*

interaction with other students any infestations may be localized and not spread. Added to this debate is the question of who is qualified to diagnose head lice. There may be volunteers available in the community. Final diagnosis should be made by a qualified professional. Each school administration must make the choice on whether head lice checks are appropriate for their building. The child's privacy, training of the head lice staff, and basic education should be of high priority in any head lice management plan.

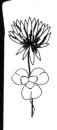

Important Message for **ADULTS** !

Many consider the most harmful effect of head lice to be the result of our response. Children often feel anxiety, fear and loss of self-esteem when confronted with head lice.

Culturally there is a stigma attached to lice that needs to be eliminated. The author hopes this book sheds some light on this issue.

RESOURCES:

- *www.cdc.gov/lice/head/treatment.html Centers for Disease Control and Prevention site contains guidelines and treatment options.*

- *www.headlice.org by the National Pediculosis Association®, Inc.*

- *www.headliceinfo.com American Head Lice Information Center*

- *Head Lice to Dead Lice by Joan Sawyer and Roberta MacPhee, St. Martin's Paperbacks, 1999. Excellent book for adults interested in the olive oil treatment plan.*

- *www.hsph.harvard.edu/headlice.html. Information and Frequently Asked Questions by Richard J. Pollack, PhD , Harvard School of Public Health, contains good photos of louse and nits.*

- *www.michigan.gov/documents Final_Michigan_Head_Lice _Manual_Michigan Head Lice Manual: A comprehensive guide to identify, treat, manage and prevent head lice written by the Michigan Department of Community Health and the Michigan Department of Education.*

- *www.oakgov.com/health/assets/documents/fs_headlice Public Health Fact Sheet: Head Lice and Household Checklist: The Lousy Work Pamphlets by the Oakland County Michigan Health Division Department of Health & Human Services*

- *www.DawQuin.com The publisher's website contains links to resources.*

- *Check with your local, county, or state health department. Some even provide diagnosis, medicated shampoos, and nit combs.*

Get It Next:

CLOVER'S **BIG** PROBLEM

Written and Illustrated by: B. L. Dawson

Can you guess which character is overweight? Why? Book #2 promises to be another fact filled entertaining story.

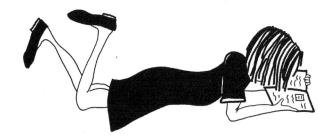

 Clover Series of Tender Teaching™

To place orders:

Go to www.DawQuin.com